The Silent Pandemic in America
Autoimmune Disease

Action Plan & Interventions for Healthcare Practitioners

Dr. Lisa Marie Portugal, PhD, EdD
The Leadership Architect

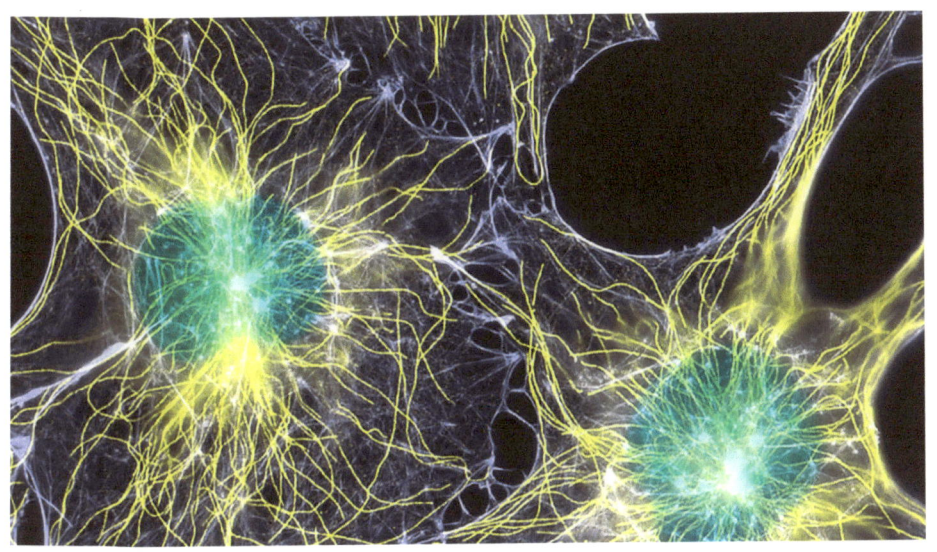

**The Silent Pandemic in America Autoimmune Disease
Action Plan & Interventions for Healthcare Practitioners**

Copyright © November 29, 2020 by Dr. Lisa Marie Portugal, PhD, EdD
All rights reserved under copyright conventions.
Published in the United States by Dr. Lisa Marie Portugal, PhD, EdD
The Leadership Architect

Library of Congress Cataloguing-in-Publication data is available
ISBN 979-8574056769
Printed in the United States
First Edition

Table of Contents

Abstract	7
Keywords	8
Chelation IV Therapy	10
Introduction	11
Example of a Health Needs Assessment	17
Needs Assessment & Intervention Mapping	23
A Health Education & Intervention Program Program Objectives & Goals	27
Action Plan & Interventions	29
Major Autohemotherapy	37
Program Evaluators	43
Project Management Strategy	43
Monitoring & Evaluating	47
Conclusion	50
About the Author	51

Contact 52

References 53

Disclaimer 60

Are you, your child, family members, or friends damaged by vaccines? This book will help you understand the research regarding heavy metals damage and autoimmune diseases. The good news is there is hope & you can get help! Chelation IV intravenous therapy & naturopathy medicine can remove heavy metals, damaging toxins, and carcinogens. Research where you can find a naturopathy doctor, integrative medicine doctor, functional medicine doctor, or holistic clinic in your area who can fully evaluate the health problem and develop a plan of action for healing. To remove heavy metals from the body, you must find an integrative doctor to do Chelation therapy. Allopathic doctors are not certified in this area and cannot do Chelation.

Tissues of The Body Affected By Autoimmune Attack

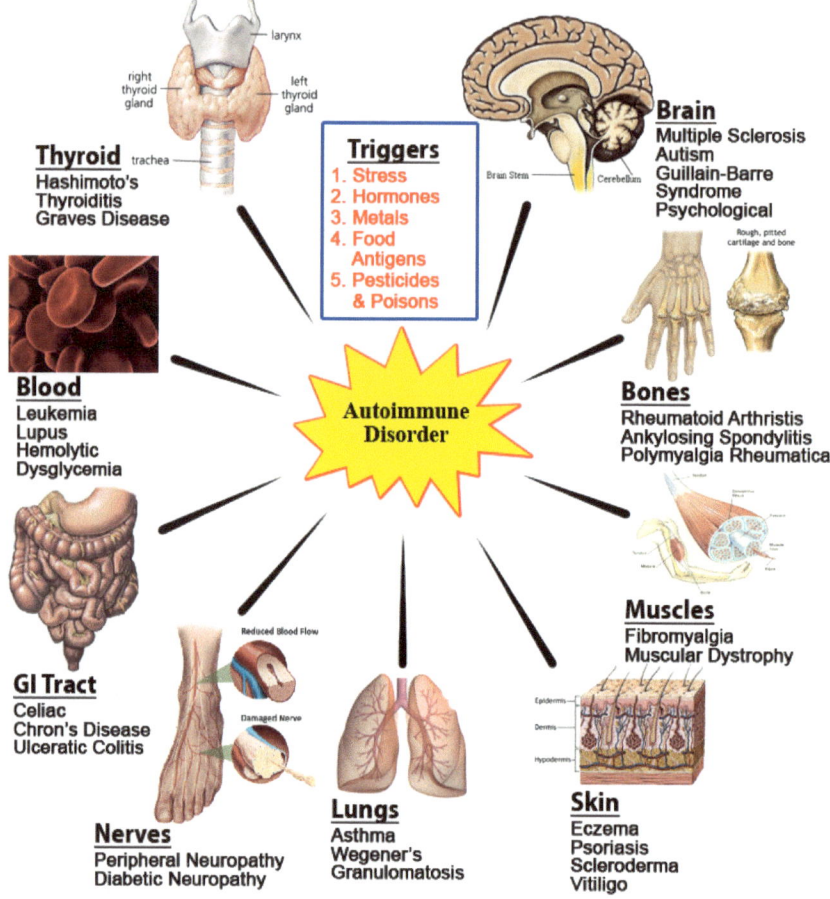

Adapted from cs@carbswitch.com (2015, February 9). *What is autoimmune disease.* https://carbswitch.com/2015/02/09/what-is-autoimmune-disease

Abstract

The book examines a health pandemic affecting a growing number of individuals in the United States. Health problems related to a needs assessment include baseline data collected from research journal articles and other health related agencies. The health pandemic is prioritized by identifying target populations in the United States who have been affected by Autoimmune Diseases and high levels of inflammation (Afeltra, Abbate, Valentini, & Giacomelli, 2019; Duan, Rao, & Sigdel, 2019; Long, Wang, Chen, Wang, Zhao, & Lu, 2018; NIAID, 2017; Rayman, 2019). A needs assessment can be administered to target populations via small groups, in-person, in-clinic, or online consultations as well as online curriculum modules.

ISBN: 9798574056769

Cover image: MIT Department of Biology. (20196). *Cell biology.* https://biology.mit.edu/faculty-and-research/areas-of-research/cell-biology/

Keywords: Vaccine Damage, Autoimmune Disease, Heavy Metals, Poisoning, Arsenic, Cadmium, Chelating agent, Copper, Iron, Lead, Mercury, Metal Toxicity, Pandemic, Epidemic, Epidemiology, Epidemiologist, Health Education, Intervention Program, Implement, Monitor, Evaluate, Program Evaluation, United States, Diagnosis, Allopathic, Pharmaceutical, Integrative Medicine, Functional Medicine, Immune System, Chelation Therapy, IV Nutrient Therapies, Lupus Erythematosus, Type 1 Diabetes, Type 2 Diabetes, Inflammatory Bowel Disease, Rheumatoid Arthritis, Environmental Exposures, Pollutants, Infections, Balance Ph, Agricultural Chemicals, Pesticides, Glyphosate, Vitamin D, Vitamin C, B12, Homeopathic, Naturopathy, Health Disparities, Needs Assessment, Intervention Mapping, Intervention Program, Colon Hydrotherapy, Colonics, Nutritional IV's, Mercury Poisoning, Lead Poisoning, Arsenic Poisoning, Cadmium Poisoning, Microbiome, Leaky Gut, Process Evaluation, Impact Evaluation, Outcome Evaluation.

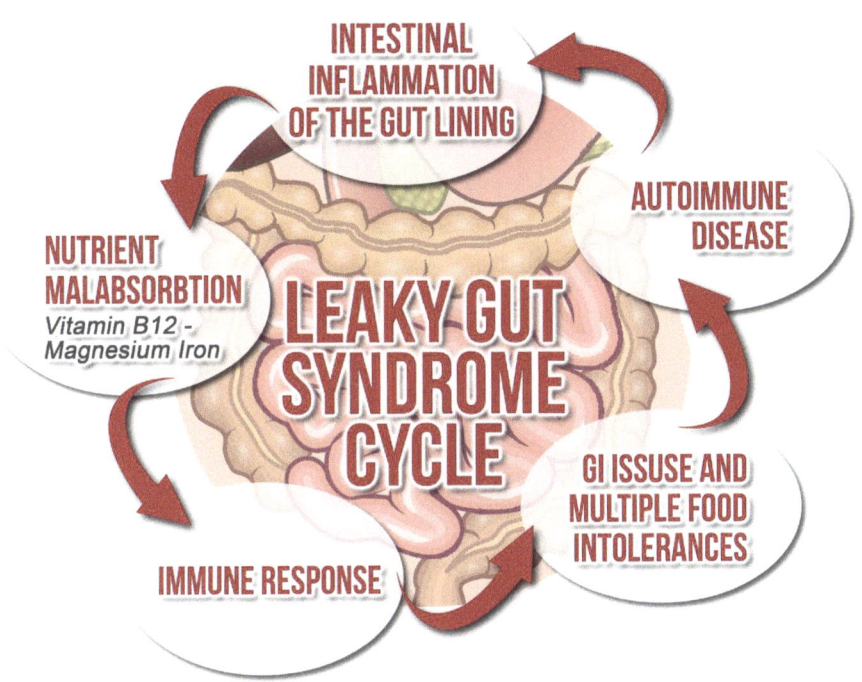

Adapted from Revived Life Health and Wellness. (n.d.). *Leaky gut: What is leaky gut.* https://revivedlife.net/leaky-gut/

Chelation IV Therapy

Chelation therapy is an extremely effective therapeutic for removing heavy metals from the body, aiding in the repair of arteries damaged by chemicals in the bloodstream, and removing excess calcium (CNIM; 2019). Chelation is best known for treating heavy metal poisoning, although it can also be used as a treatment for circulatory disorders and heart disease (CNIM; 2019). Furthermore, chelation therapy enhances the body's ability to flow blood more efficiently and easily (CNIM; 2019). Chelation has afforded patients a successful and effective manner to heal heart disease rather than invasive harmful heart surgery (CNIM; 2019). Chelation can be used as a treatment to avoid limb amputation for diabetics, reduce high blood pressure, and alleviate angina (CNIM; 2019). With an impeccable record of safety, and over the last 50 years, many suffering individuals chose chelation for a broad spectrum of circulatory health challenges (CNIM, 2019). "A review of 40 published and 30 unpublished studies involving over 25,000 patients who underwent EDTA chelation demonstrated that 87 percent benefited from this therapy (CNIM, 2019).

The Silent Pandemic in America
Autoimmune Disease

Introduction

The book explains program objectives and goals for a health education and intervention program for autoimmune disease patients. In addition, a comprehensive project management intervention strategy and implementation plan is summarized. How to monitor and evaluate the intervention plan is described. Finally, the role of program evaluators is addressed. Graphics are included throughout the book.

Autoimmune disease is a health pandemic affecting many individuals in the United States (AARDA, 2020; NIAID, 2017). Major obstacles related to the health problem include: (1) diagnosis is difficult, (2) understanding about the health problem by allopathic doctors is limited, and (3) understanding how to heal the health problem is difficult when practitioners do not have the knowledge or training necessary to address the problem (AARDA, 2020). Symptoms related to Autoimmune disease intersect many specialties and can affect every organ in the human body. Allopathic medical training offers minimal education regarding the health pandemic (AARDA, 2020). Allopathic providers are commonly uninformed of interrelationships between various autoimmune diseases (AARDA, 2020). In addition, practitioners trained in the allopathic business model are unaware of treatment advances that are not known throughout various specialty areas (AARDA, 2020). Typically, beginning symptoms can be unspecific and intermittent before the disease advances to an acute stage (AARDA, 2020; NIAID, 2017). Additional challenges such as a limited amount of research conducted on the topic is typically limited in scope and disease-specific (AARDA, 2020; NIAID, 2017). This challenge adds to the misinformed and uneducated nature of allopathic practitioners (AARDA, 2020). Furthermore, an increased crossover between research projects and information sharing regarding various autoimmune diseases is necessary (AARDA, 2020).

Different Types of Autoimmune Disease Disorders

AUTOIMMUNE DISEASES

Brain
Multiple Sclerosis
Guillain-Barre Syndrome
Autism

Thyroid
Thyroiditis
Hashimoto's Disease
Graves' Disease

Blood
Leukemia
Lupus Erythematosus
Hemolytic Dysglycemia

Bones
Rheumatoid Arthritis
Ankylosing Spondylitis
Polymyalgia Rheumatica

GI Tract
Celiac's Disease
Crohn's Disease
Ulcerative Colitis
Diabetes Type I

Muscles
Rheumatoid Arthritis
Ankylosing Spondylitis
Polymyalgia Rheumatica

Nerves
Peripheral Neuropathy
Diabetic Neuropathy

Skin
Psoriasis
Vitiligo
Eczema
Scleroderma

Lung
Fibromyalgia
Wegener's Granulomatosis

Over 100 Different Types of AutoImmune Disorders

Adapted from DrJockers.com (n.d.). *The 7 major factors causing autoimmune conditions.* https://drjockers.com/7-factors-causing-autoimmune-conditions/

Autoimmune disease is a significant health pandemic and spans throughout many races, cultures, and groups within in the United States (NIAID, 2017). Clustering of the disease can be found in families and groups of individuals with close relationships and similar lifestyle choices and dietary habits (NIAID, 2017).

Knowledgeable and educated health practitioners are needed who understand how to balance immune system activity and who can address the health pandemic. More research is needed in this area to educate health practitioners and the public regarding how to heal the body and raise immunity through integrative, holistic, and functional medicine practices such as Chelation and IV nutrient therapies to remove heavy metals as well as targeted diet and nutrition remedies (Konijeti, Kim, Lewis, Groven, Chandrasekaran, Grandhe, Diamant, Singh, Oliveira, Wang, Molparia, & Torkamani, 2017). Health discoveries in these areas and practices have made autoimmune research an encouraging area for new discovery (NIAID, 2017).

According to the National Institute of Allergy and Infectious Disease (NIAID), the debilitating and chronic complexity of these vast array of diseases result in a diminished quality of life and rising medical costs causing burdens on patients, families, and communities. Reports indicate that more than 80 diseases develop because of the body's immune system assaulting its own tissues, organs, and cells (NIAID, 2017). Frequent autoimmune diseases consist of systemic lupus erythematosus, type 1 diabetes, inflammatory bowel disease, and rheumatoid arthritis (Afeltra et al., 2019; Duan et al., 2019; Long et al., 2018; NIAID, 2017; Rayman, 2019). Other autoimmune diseases are more difficult to diagnose (NIEHS, 2020). Many autoimmune diseases are caused by toxic environmental exposures and infections (NIAID, 2017). Additionally, herbicides such as Monsanto's Glyphosate in the food supply, high levels of heavy metals in the body, and poor diet lacking nutritional benefits to raise immunity and balance Ph are other variables negatively affecting individuals dealing with autoimmune diseases (Konijeti et al., 2017).

Patients commonly suffer years before being diagnosed with an autoimmune disease and allopathic providers do not know how to cure or heal these diseases (NIEHS, 2020). Commonly, allopathic practitioners prescribe lifelong pharmaceutical treatments only in an effort to manage some symptoms. In the United States, autoimmune diseases collectively affect more than 24 million individuals and an additional eight million with auto-antibodies blood molecules indicating a high prediction for developing autoimmune disease (NIEHS, 2020). According to beliefs held in the allopathic business model, autoimmune diseases are affecting more individuals for unknown reasons (NIEHS, 2020). Moreover, the causes of these diseases continue to be a mystery to allopathic providers (NIEHS, 2020). According to the National Institute of Environmental Health Sciences (2020), autoimmune diseases tend to be more common when the following environmental exposures are present:

- Agricultural chemicals and pesticides,
- Mercury exposure,
- Environmental pollutants, and
- A multitude of diet and nutrition problems leading to a lack of important vitamins and nutrients such as Vitamin D and many others (NIEHS, 2020).

Dietary micronutrients have been found to improve the health of patients with autoimmune diseases (NIEHS, 2020).

Since most allopathic providers have not been properly educated and trained regarding autoimmune diseases, inflammation (NIAID, 2017), and diet and nutritional medicine, also called functional medicine, practitioners in the allopathic business model do not have the tools, knowledge, or the certification to address these problems. Chelation and IV nutrient therapies require homeopathic and naturopathy certification to legally administer and practice. Most allopathic providers are lacking the board certified credentials and medical training in this area of medicine. In addition, allopathic providers believe there are no cures (NIAID, 2017) and commonly prescribe unnecessary pharmaceutical drugs that cause many additional harmful side effects. Allopathic practitioners have not been trained (NIAID, 2017) or certified to understand what causes autoimmune diseases or how to heal the pandemic facing a vast number of Americans. Treatments are available for many autoimmune diseases that do not involve harmful, toxic pharmaceutical drugs or unnecessary surgery. Healing can be found through integrative, holistic, functional medical practitioners who are knowledgeable, educated, and certified to address and heal autoimmune diseases.

Example of a Health Needs Assessment in Relation to its Purpose

Health practitioners conduct a needs assessment to aid in identifying gaps in services and resources in areas where groups and individuals in a community might be at a greater risk for poor health outcomes and health disparities. Data related to health behaviors and outcomes, access to health services, socioeconomic status, and demographics can provide a more comprehensive understanding of the assets and needs of communities (Bartholomew, Markham, Ruiter, Fernàndez, Kok, & Parcel, 2016; Kok, Gottlieb, Peters, Mullen, Parcel, Ruiter, Fernández, Markham, & Bartholomew, 2016). Public health policymakers and change agents can use a needs assessment tool to determine developing health challenges, to identify hard-to-reach or hidden populations, and to identify where individuals are not obtaining services to address health needs (Bartholomew et al., 2016; Kok et al., 2016). As a foundation, health practitioners can use the strengths of a community to aid in improving health for target populations. An example of how healthcare practitioners can use a needs assessment could involve addressing the pandemic of autoimmune diseases in the United States.

Needs Assessment Methods

Needs Assessment Methods

Method	Kinds of Data	Good for ?	Features	Specific Uses
Surveys	•Opinions, •Preferences •Self-report of behavior •Easily analyzed as quantitative information	•Aggregate information •Big picture •Comparison of sub-groups (if sufficient #s)	•Cheap •Challenging to design well •Difficult to get high enough response rate to ensure validity	Identify: •Interest in topics •Prioritization •Levels of satisfaction •Stakeholder information
Interviews	•Opinions, •Preferences •Informed, thoughtful •Qualitative	•Expert input •Details, rationale •Triangulation	•Labor, time intensive •Permit interactive probing	•Identify: •Explanatory details, esp. post-survey •Vested interests of stakeholders

Adapted from Milne, L. (2009, June 25). *Needs assessment.*
https://www.slideshare.net/lynda.milne/needs-assessment-1638514

How Metal Toxicity Affects the Body

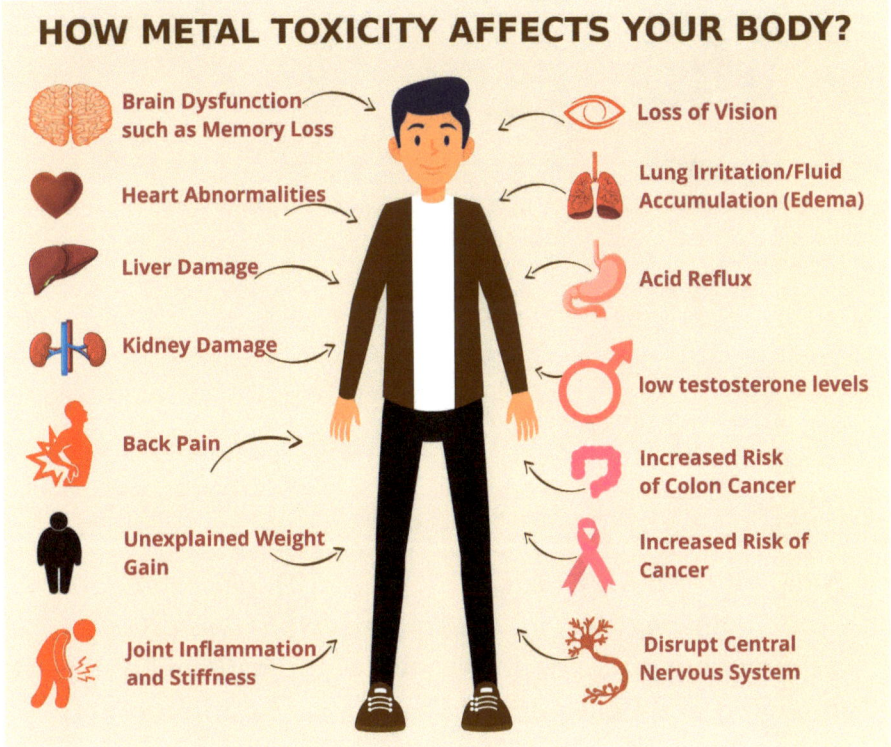

Adapted from Daivam Wellness (2019, October 16). *When was the last time your doctor asked you to take a metal toxicity test?* https://www.daivamwellness.com/when-was-the-last-time-your-doctor-asked-you-to-take-a-metal-toxicity-test/

Molar Teeth with Heavy Metal Fillings

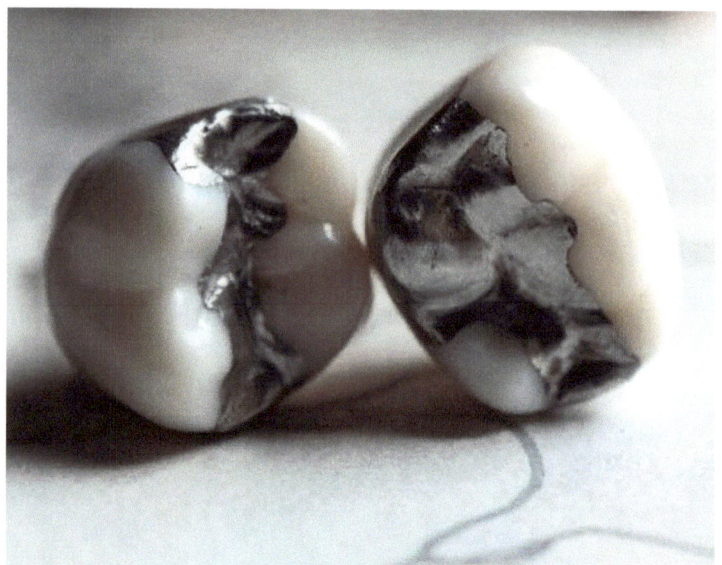

Adapted from Maja, J. (2019, April 10). *How amalgam (and heavy metals) can cause Hashimoto and other autoimmune diseases.* https://www.joannamaja.com/how-amalgam-and-heavy-metals-can-cause-hashimoto-and-other-autoimmune-diseases/

Glyphosate Gluten Intolerant Pandemic

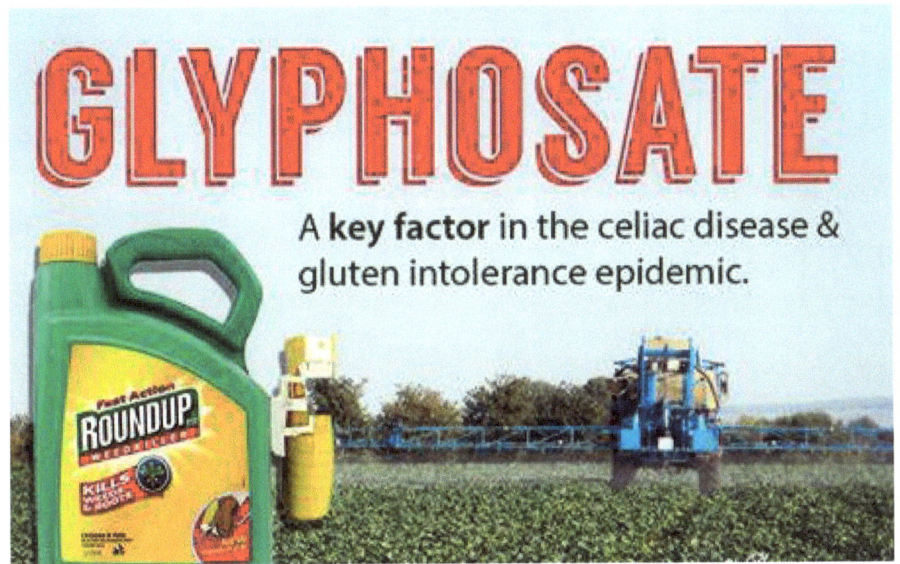

Adapted from Redoubt News LLC & Granny Good Food (2017, July 7). *Gluten intolerance is really GLYPHOSATE POISONING.* https://redoubtnews.com/2017/07/gluten-monsanto-glyphosate-poisoning/

Glyphosate Applied to Wheat 1990 to 2010

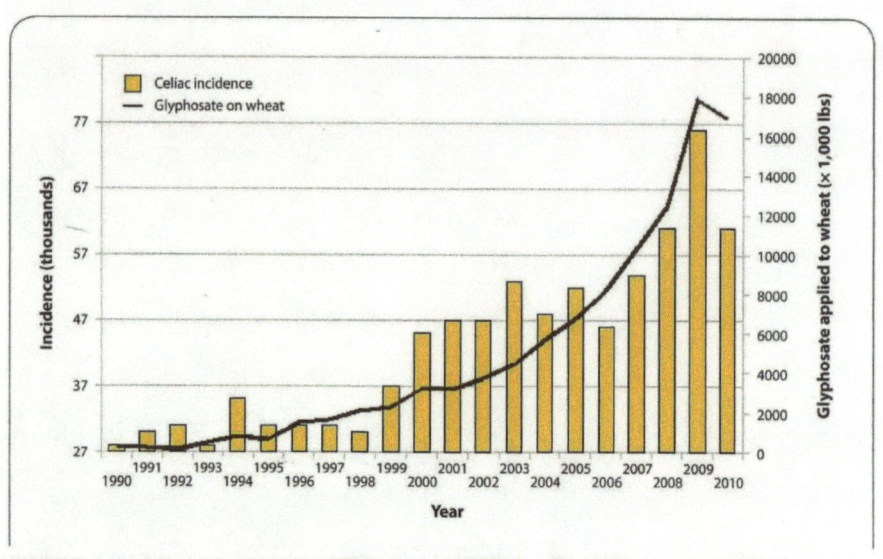

Adapted from Redoubt News LLC & Granny Good Food (2017, July 7). *Gluten intolerance is really GLYPHOSATE POISONING.* https://redoubtnews.com/2017/07/gluten-monsanto-glyphosate-poisoning/

How a Needs Assessment is connected to the Process of Intervention Mapping

A needs assessment can involve the use of intervention mapping to aid in identifying health challenges and disparities within a community or target population. Intervention mapping involves the following key steps:

- Conducting a problem analysis or needs assessment.
- Identifying what needs to be changed.
- Determining who needs intervention.
- Creating change matrices with targets linking:
- Secondary behaviors and performance targets with behavioral determinants, and
- Determining beliefs that need to be addressed by a behavioral mediation.
- Choosing intervention methods based on theory with matching behavioral determinants.
- Targeting beliefs that have been identified.
- Translating into practical applications that help target populations and individuals make positive behavioral health changes.
- Incorporating methods and practical applications into a coordinated health intervention program.
- Preparing for choosing, implementing, and sustaining a health intervention initiative in real-life situations.

- Developing assessment methods to conduct process and effect assessments (Bartholomew et al., 2016; Kok et al., 2016).

The Intervention Mapping Process

Intervention Mapping Process*

Step 1: Conduct Needs Assessment
Step 2: Specify Change Objectives
Step 3: Select Theory-based Methods & Practical Strategies
Step 4: Develop Program Components
Step 5: Specify Adoption & Implementation
Step 6: Generate Evaluation Plan

* Bartholomew, Parcel, Kok, Gottlieb, 2001; 2nd Edition. 2006

Adapted from Mcleod, B. (n.d.). *Introduction to intervention mapping - PowerPoint PPT presentation.* https://www.slideserve.com/benedict/introduction-to-intervention-mapping

The key to lasting healing is knowing the right information and the right healers, doctors, and scientific researchers. Wisdom is life changing and saves lives. In addition, turning off the fear-based Big corporate media and learning about how one can take personal action in his or her life to create a lifestyle of healing and change rather than a lifestyle of weakness, dependency thinking, fear, and misinformation is critical to health and wellbeing.

AUTOIMMUNE DISEASES

- Lupus
- multiple sclerosis
- type 1 diabetes
- rheumatoid arthritis
- Parkinson's
- Fibromyalgia
- Chronic Fatigue Syndrome
- ASD's ???
- nearly a hundred other known autoimmune diseases.

autoimmune diseases
- One in 12 people
- one in 9 women
- 24 million Americans
- double the number of people who have cancer
- woman is 8 times more likely to have an autoimmune disease than breast cancer
- 90 percent of Americans say they can't name a single autoimmune disease

Foods That Heal
Foods That Kill

"Let food be your medicine and medicine be your food" Hippocrates

"Anything you take in your body will make you either Healthier or Sicker" Dr. Bergman

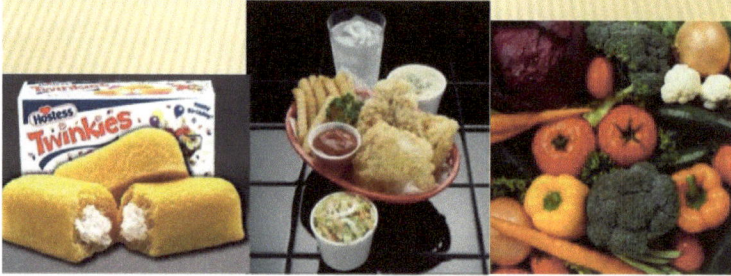

Adapted from Bergman, J. (2015, April 15). *Auto immune disease 2015*. https://www.slideshare.net/johnbchiro/auto-immune-disease-2015

A Health Education & Intervention Program for Autoimmune Disease Patients

Program Objectives & Goals

Health educators and shareholders can design program interventions that benefit changes in health behavior, health literacy, and overall health and wellbeing of patients with autoimmune disease. A comprehensive health education and promotion program for autoimmune patients can involve the following components:

- Interpreting and analyzing multiple and comprehensive collected health data concerning interests and needs in cultural and social environments.
- Differentiating behaviors that hinder and foster well-being.
- Determining essential requirements needed for a health education intervention based upon data obtained.
- Gathering, analyzing, describing, and reporting information regarding disease, health, and delivery of healthcare services.
- Selecting and recruiting shareholders.
- Constructing logical sequence and scope plan.
- Formulating measurable objectives.
- Executing the plan.

- Selecting media and methods appropriate for the plan.
- Analyzing and revising the plan as needed.
- Selecting and using counseling techniques and adjusting for individualized needs of patients.
- Assessing program achievements and objectives.
- Interpreting results.
- Inferring implications for future program planning (Bartholomew, Markham, Ruiter, Fernàndez, Kok, & Parcel, 2016; Fernandez, Ruiter, Markham, & Kok, 2019; Goudet, Murira, Torlesse, Hatchard, & Busch-Hallen, 2018; Kok, Gottlieb, Peters, Mullen, Parcel, Ruiter, Fernández, Markham, & Bartholomew, 2016).

The role of affective and learning experiences is critical in health education, promotion, and behavioral change (Bartholomew et al., 2016; Fernandez et al., 2019; Goudet et al., 2018; Kok et al., 2016). Self-evaluation and self-motivation is integral in strengthening experiential learning opportunities (Bartholomew et al., 2016; Fernandez et al., 2019; Goudet et al., 2018; Kok et al., 2016). The trust and confidentiality of patients suffering from autoimmune disorders can be established by health educators and shareholders maintaining a scrupulous *do no harm* code of ethics that notoriously and consistently has been lacking in the allopathic and pharmaceutical business model.

Action Plan & Interventions for Autoimmune Patients

Before starting any intervention, the integrative medical team of health practitioners involved in the healing process must conduct a full medical evaluation for each patient, which includes obtaining full medical records, blood work, and interviewing the patient in detail. The interviews must involve questions pertaining to what the patient puts on the body, in the body, and what the patient is surrounded by in his or her daily environment to assess diet, physical activity, toxins in the environment, and deficiencies that may need to be addressed in the intervention. Once a full medical assessment has been conducted, the integrative medical team of health practitioners can develop an individualized intervention plan based upon the patient's needs and deficiencies that must be addressed.

Various symptoms exhibited by patients with autoimmune disease can include, but are not limited to, irritability and stress, chronic pain, menstrual disorders, headaches, digestive issues, and chronic disease.

Essential elements of healing autoimmune disease can include colon hydrotherapy to:

- eliminate chronic constipation;
- aid the body to facilitate waste elimination;
- aid the body to increase energy;

- aid the body to detoxify; and
- aid the body to reduce cravings for sugar addiction and other unhealthy processed food cravings (Fontes & Stawicki, n.d.).

Colon hydrotherapy can aid with the following symptoms:

- frequent illness,
- pain in joints,
- low-back pain,
- gas,
- bad breath,
- body odor,
- chronic fatigue,
- bags under the eyes,
- inability to sleep,
- depression,
- brain fog,
- thyroid disruption,
- diabetes,
- migraines,
- stress,
- hormonal imbalance,
- constipation, and
- weight gain (Fontes & Stawicki, n.d.).

A colon that is unhealthy strains the kidneys and overloads liver function (Fontes & Stawicki, n.d.). Toxicity builds up and creates additional health challenges (Fontes & Stawicki, n.d.). A colonic protocol is a safe and effective way to eliminate waste and toxins from the body without harmful pharmaceutical drugs (Fontes & Stawicki, n.d.). In addition, unblocking Qi-energy flow in the body by facilitating detoxification with acupuncture aids the body in healing (Fontes & Stawicki, n.d.). In addition, unblocking Qi-energy flow in the body by facilitating detoxification with acupuncture aids the body in healing (Fontes & Stawicki, n.d.).

Unhealthy Colon versus Healthy Colon

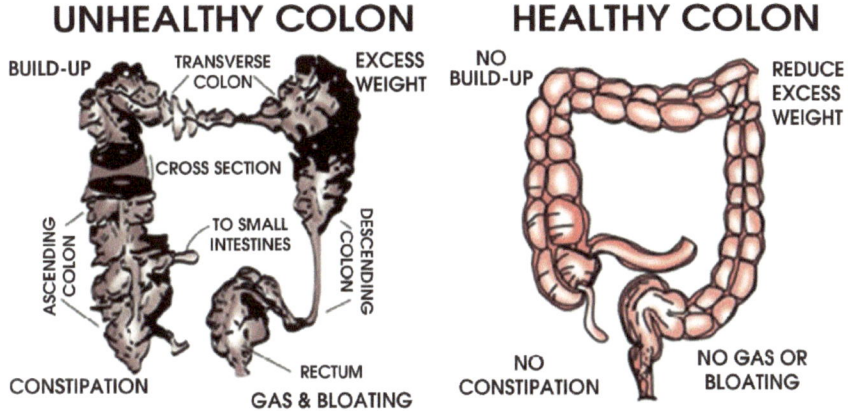

Adapted from Fontes, M., & Stawicki, M. (n.d.). *Natural medicine and detox.* https://naturalmedicineanddetox.com/

Remedies to aid in detoxification and raising the body's immunity can include intravenous (IV) therapies such as:

- Vitamin C IV therapy heals and promotes immunity;
- Ultraviolet blood irradiation cleans blood of bacteria, fungus, and virus;
- Ozone therapy heals and promotes immunity;
- Myers' cocktail IV therapy provides the body with essential vitamins and minerals;
- Hydrogen peroxide IV therapy cleans the body of bacteria, fungus, and virus;
- Chelation IV therapy removes heavy metals (CNIM, 2019; Kim, Kim, & Kumar, 2019; Osborne & Anderson, 2007);
- B-12 injections heal and promote immunity; and
- Nutritional IV's provides the body with essential vitamins and minerals lacking in diet (Fontes & Stawicki, n.d.).

Common metal poisoning can include mercury, lead, cadmium, and arsenic. Toxic heavy metals can be absorbed by the body through:

- environmental factors,
- industrial exposure,
- water pollution,
- pharmaceuticals and allopathic medicines,
- X-ray machines, and
- plastic food containers, pots, and pans improperly coated with toxic manufactured materials (CNIM, 2019; Kim, Kim, & Kumar, 2019; GARD, 2017; Gotter & Murrell, 2018).

General symptoms of heavy metal poisoning can include, but are not limited to, the following:

- full body or some parts of the body in chronic pain,
- joint pain,
- dizziness or vertigo,
- exhaustion, feeling tired all the time, low energy,
- shortness of breath,
- tingling in hands and feet,
- nausea,
- abdominal pain,
- diarrhea,
- chills,
- weakness, and
- vomiting (CNIM, 2019; Kim, Kim, & Kumar, 2019; GARD, 2017; Gotter & Murrell, 2018).

Mercury poisoning symptoms can include:

- trouble walking,
- vision changes,
- nerve damage in feet and hands,
- speech and hearing difficulties,
- weakness in muscles, and
- lack of coordination (CNIM, 2019; Kim, Kim, & Kumar, 2019; GARD, 2017; Gotter & Murrell, 2018).

Lead poisoning symptoms can include:

- loss of developmental skills in children,
- memory loss,
- fatigue,
- headaches,
- anemia,
- loss of appetite,
- high blood pressure,
- irritability,
- sleep problems,
- aggressive behavior, and
- constipation (CNIM, 2019; Kim, Kim, & Kumar, 2019; GARD, 2017; Gotter & Murrell, 2018).

Arsenic poisoning symptoms can include:

- muscle cramps,
- unusual heart rhythm,
- spots on skis such as lesions and warts,
- swollen or red skin, and
- diarrhea, vomiting, or nausea (CNIM, 2019; Kim, Kim, & Kumar, 2019; GARD, 2017; Gotter & Murrell, 2018).

Cadmium poisoning symptoms can include:

- muscle pain,
- breathing problems, and
- fever (CNIM, 2019; Kim, Kim, & Kumar, 2019; GARD, 2017; Gotter & Murrell, 2018).

Chelation therapy is an extremely effective therapeutic for removing heavy metals from the body, aiding in the repair of arteries damaged by chemicals in the bloodstream, and removing excess calcium (CNIM; 2019). Chelation is best known for treating heavy metal poisoning, although it can also be used as a treatment for circulatory disorders and heart disease (CNIM; 2019). Furthermore, chelation therapy enhances the body's ability to flow blood more efficiently and easily (CNIM; 2019). Chelation has afforded patients a successful and effective manner to heal heart disease rather than invasive harmful heart surgery (CNIM; 2019).

Furthermore, chelation can be used as a treatment to avoid limb amputation for diabetics, reduce high blood pressure, and alleviate angina (CNIM; 2019).

Chelation therapy can benefit the following conditions:

- Peripheral vascular disease,
- Intermittent claudication,
- Diabetic complications,
- Peripheral neuropathy,

- Hypertension,
- Cerebrovascular disease,
- Slow healing wounds,
- Memory disorders,
- Detoxification therapies for heavy metals, and
- Cardiovascular disease (CNIM, 2019).

With an impeccable record of safety, and over the last 50 years, many suffering individuals chose chelation for a broad spectrum of circulatory health challenges (CNIM, 2019). "A review of 40 published and 30 unpublished studies involving over 25,000 patients who underwent EDTA chelation demonstrated that 87 percent benefited from this therapy (CNIM, 2019).

Major Autohemotherapy (MAH)

Other ways to kill pathogens in the body include ultra violet blood irradiation therapy and ozone therapy, which involve therapies that add oxygen and ozone to the blood and passing the blood through an ultra violet light to kill viruses, parasites, fungus, and bacteria. These therapies aid in healing many chronic autoimmune diseases and autism. Find a holistic clinic, naturopathy doctor, or integrative doctor in your area and ask about these life-changing therapies.

"Major Autohemotherapy (or MAH) is a type of IV therapy in which your blood is first withdrawn from your vein into an IV bag, and then mixed with medical ozone. After your blood and ozone are mixed together in the bag, the mixture will be dripped back into your vein. As a result, no Ozone actually enters your bloodstream. Rather the biological byproduct of the external mixing of your blood with ozone (ozinides, etc.) are actually creating the healing effect" (Tringali-Health.com (2020).

- Ozone improves mitochondrial function and efficiency.
- Ozone makes red blood cells more elastic and flexible.
- Ozone kills bacteria, fungi, mold, and viruses.
- Ozone stimulates the production of Tumor necrosis Factor.

- Ozone stimulates increased levels of Interferon levels.
- Ozone stimulates the production of white blood cells (Tringali-Health.com (2020).

MAH can be used as a therapy for the following health problems:

- Tinnitus (vascular only)
- Acute hearing loss (vascular only)
- Low Immunity
- Infections (viral, bacterial, fungal)
- Eye Diseases especially retinopathies
- (shingles)
- Herpes simplex and herpes zoster
- Hepatitis B and C
- Asthma and COPD
- Diabetic Circulatory Disease
- Post Stroke
- Dementia and Cerebral Vascular Disease
- Peripheral Artery Disease
- Heart and Vascular Disease
- Auto Immune Disease
- Osteo and Rheumatoid Arthritis
- LYME Disease
- Chronic Allergies
- Chemical Sensitivities
- Fibromyalgia
- Chronic Fatigue and CF

- Autism (Tringali-Health.com (2020).

Five essential elements for successful detox include the following:

1. drainage,
2. elimination,
3. nutrition,
4. inflammation, and
5. detoxification (Fontes & Stawicki, n.d.).

Healing the body's microbiome is essential because 60% of the body's immunity is in the intestinal track. Healing a *leaky gut* related to pesticides and Glyphosate poisoning in the food supply is essential to a healthy microbiome. Knowledgeable integrative healthcare practitioners can educate patients and explain how this type of healing is accomplished. Furthermore, addressing diet, nutrition, and essential vitamins and minerals lacking in the patient's profile must be targeted factors in an individualized intervention plan to heal autoimmune disease.

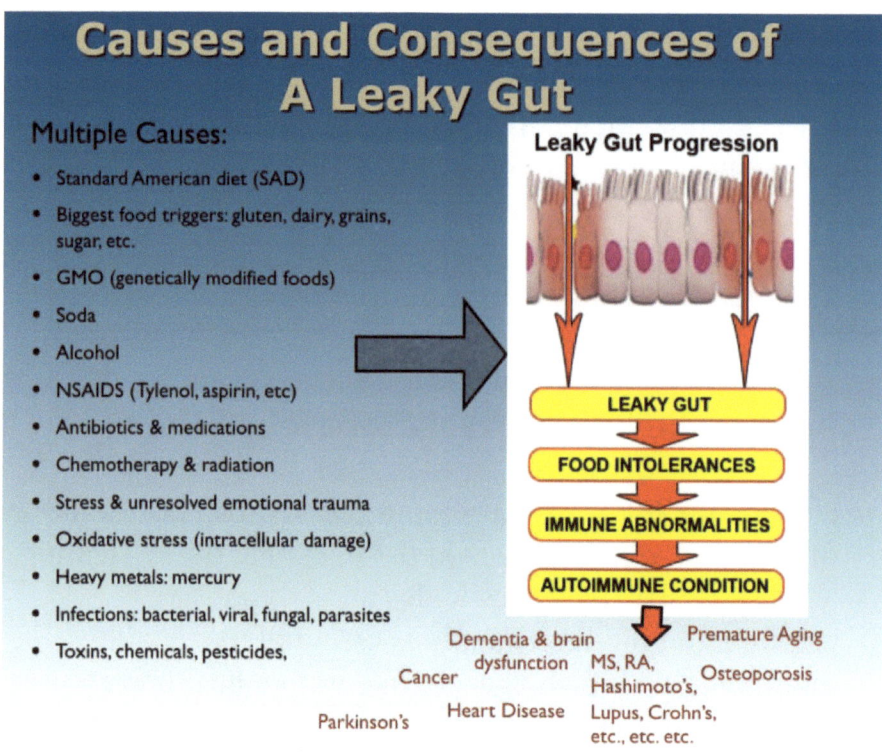

Adapted from Five Seasons Functional Medicine. (2019). *What is intestinal permeability (leaky gut)?* https://fiveseasonsmedical.com/leaky-gut/

Key areas that must be included in a personalized intervention plan involve aiding the body's elimination processes by detoxing heavy metals, waste, toxins, and pesticides with targeted and integrative therapies. Moreover, the integrative medical team will address building the body's immunity based upon what essential vitamins and minerals are lacking from the patient's diet by prescribing a specific nutrition regime, herbs, plants, roots, fruits, nuts, and spices with targeted individualized integrative therapeutics. A focus on education regarding probiotic foods is necessary as well. Food has the power to cure or kill. Food is medicine and can be used to build a better immune system. An integrative medical team can aid autoimmune patients in removing toxins from the body, reducing unhealthy cravings, building the body's immunity, and educating about diet and nutrition.

5 Elements of Detox

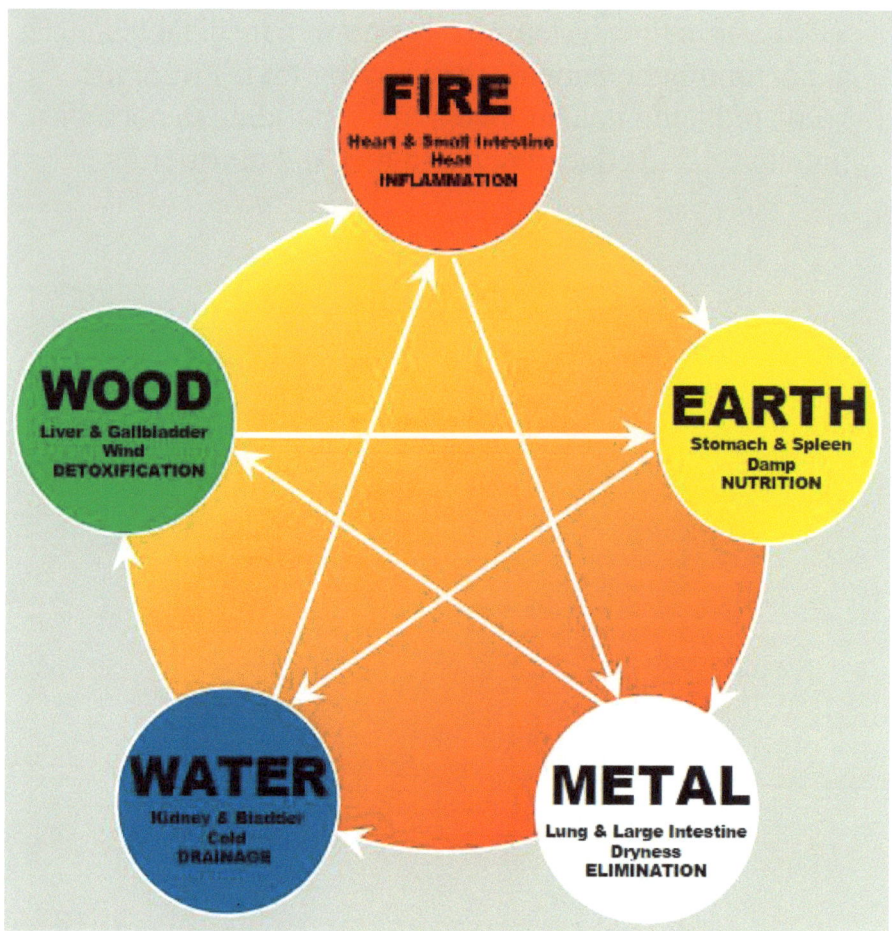

Adapted from Fontes, M., & Stawicki, M. (n.d.). *Natural medicine and detox.* https://naturalmedicineanddetox.com/

Program Evaluators

Who should evaluate? When working with autoimmune patients, various evaluators and evaluations are required. For example, participatory evaluation can involve various shareholders and activities. Primary responsibilities involve evaluation of professionalism, ethics, leadership, management, communication, advocacy, research, evaluation, implementation, planning, capacity, and needs (Lewis, 2017). Integrative health practitioners, health educators, and auxiliary health providers play specific and varied roles in the participatory evaluation, diagnosis, prescribing, documenting, and follow-up procedures for patients suffering with autoimmune disease.

Project Management Intervention Strategy & Implementation

Leaders and shareholders in healthcare seek ways to strategically and continuously advance and refine processes to improve patients' overall satisfaction and experience, reduce costs, and improve patient care (Afzal & Gauthier, 2017; Hester, Auerbach, Seeff, Wheaton, Brusuelas, & Singleton, 2016; Speziale, 2015). Project management competencies in healthcare have become significantly critical from a business perspective in the healthcare sector because these aptitudes aid in controlling costs, managing risk, and improving project outcomes (Afzal & Gauthier, 2017; Hester et al., 2016;

Speziale, 2015). When project management techniques and methodologies are applied in program design, shareholders are better equipped to plan, organize, and execute tasks in a systematic manner to maximize resources and achieve tangible objectives (Afzal & Gauthier, 2017; Hester et al., 2016; Speziale, 2015).

To conduct project management in a successful manner, involving appropriate shareholders contributing in distinctive roles with specific responsibilities can be planned and executed by the following roles and duties:

- Program manager plans, manages, and executes the program by engaging shareholders.
- Program sponsor is involved in a senior leadership manner and administrates support and guidance while making essential decisions.
- Program team involves individuals contributing to the implementation of the program.
- Program shareholders involve individuals impacted by the program's outcome or those who administer and supply resources and services (Afzal & Gauthier, 2017; Hester et al., 2016; Speziale, 2015).

Health Impact Pyramid

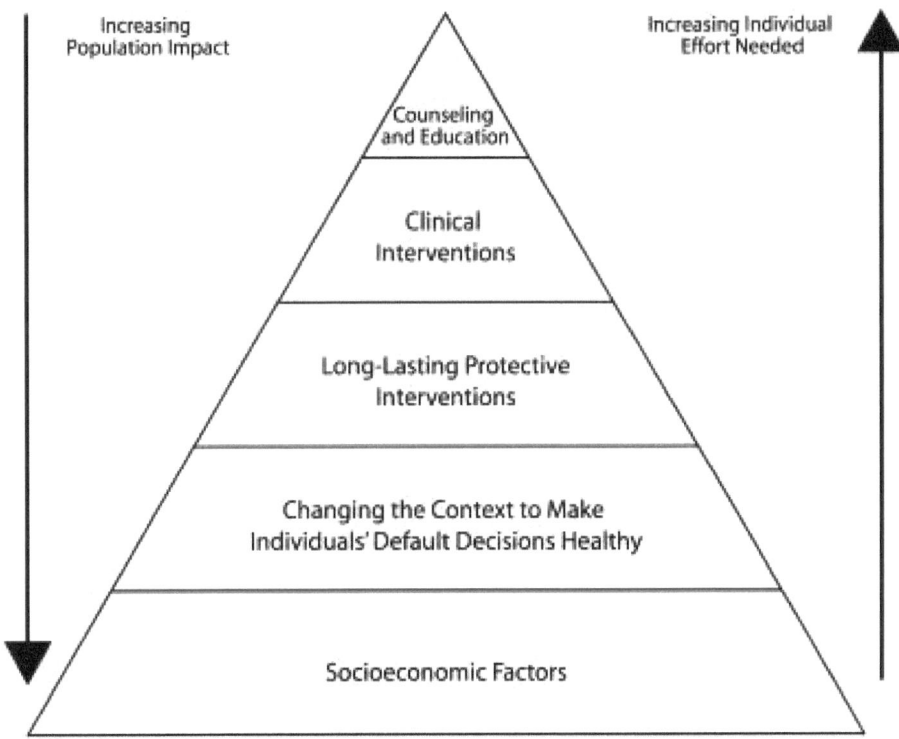

Adapted from Frieden, T. R. (2010). A framework for public health action: The health impact pyramid. *American Journal of Public Health, 100*(4), 590-595.

Phase one involves initiating the program. Phase two involves planning the program. Phase three involves executing the program. Phase four involves closing the program. Successful project management involves mindfulness of regulations, processes, privacy, quality, and patient safety (Hester et al., 2016; Speziale, 2015).

Monitoring & Evaluating the Intervention Plan

When conducting a needs assessment, it is necessary to have clarity regarding what one is evaluating, why one is evaluating, and for whom one is evaluating. These details are critical for shaping an evaluation tool that can be effective. Assessment of program effectiveness can involve three distinct processes, which include: (1) process evaluation, (2) impact evaluation, and (3) outcome evaluation (Costello, Taylor, & O'Hara, 2015; Grant, Bugge, & Wells, 2020; Jones, 2016; Sharma, van Teijlingen, Belizán, Hundley, Simkhada, & Sicuri, 2016).

Process evaluation involves the documentation and tacking of the process of a program's implementation (Grant et al., 2020). Evaluation of process aids shareholders in observing how impact and outcome of a program was accomplished (Costello et al., 2015; Goudet et al., 2018; Grant et al., 2020; Sharma et al., 2016). The objective of evaluating a process is centered on the quantities and types of:

- delivered services,
- recipients receiving services,
- resources needed in the delivery of services,
- challenges experienced, and
- whether challenges were successfully addressed and resolved (Grant et al., 2020).

Furthermore, process evaluation aids in understanding infrastructure and program management processes to decide whether the program was able to deliver its promised objectives and goals (Grant et al., 2020).

Impact evaluation involves cause-and-effect analysis using precise methods to examine outcome changes associated with specific interventions used in the program (Costello et al., 2015; Sharma et al., 2016). This type of evaluation examines what might have happened without the intervention by designing quasi-experimental or experimental studies involving treatment and comparison groups (Costello et al., 2015; Sharma et al., 2016). Impact evaluations serve to provide accountability determining how well and whether the program achieved its mission. Furthermore, impact evaluations aid in answering program design questions related to which approaches, among various that were used, were the most effective. Impact evaluations should be used:

- to test innovations in program design,
- pilot programs,
- when intervention will be replicated and scaled in other settings,
- when the intervention is untested, and
- if results of the intervention could influence important policy-making decisions (Costello et al., 2015; Sharma et al., 2016).

Outcome evaluation is commonly desired by foundations and assesses whether a program was effective in producing change. This type of evaluation queries for different questions and measures what happened to individuals participating in the program and the extent to which participation in the program affected their lives (Jones, 2016). Outcome evaluations measure program effectiveness in generating change. Process evaluations aid shareholders in understanding how a program's impact and outcome was achieved (Jones, 2016). Impact and outcome evaluations measure how well and whether objectives of the program were delivered (Costello et al., 2015; Jones, 2016; Sharma et al., 2016).

Conclusion

The book examined a health pandemic affecting a growing number of individuals in the United States. Health problems related to a needs assessment included baseline data collected from research journal articles and other health related agencies. The health pandemic was prioritized by identifying target populations in the United States who have been affected by autoimmune diseases and high levels of inflammation (Afeltra et al., 2019; Duan et al., 2019; Long et al., 2018; NIAID, 2017; Rayman, 2019).

A needs assessment can be administered to target populations via small groups, in-person, in-clinic, or online consultations as well as online curriculum modules. Furthermore, the book explained program objectives and goals for a health education and intervention program for autoimmune disease patients. In addition, a comprehensive project management intervention strategy and implementation plan was summarized. How to monitor and evaluate the intervention plan was described. Finally, the role of program evaluators was addressed. Graphics were included throughout the book.

About the Author

Dr. Lisa Marie Portugal holds a PhD in Leadership for Higher Education, MEd in Educational Business Administration Human Resources, MEd in Health and Wellness, MAEd in Secondary Education, and a BFA in Fine Arts and Media Arts. Her expertise and research interests include: health and wellness, cancer, diabetes, child and adult vaccines, Big Pharma prescription drugs, naturopathic medicine, homeopathic medicine, functional medicine, Traditional Chinese Medicine, allopathic medicine, GMO foods, pesticides, government legislation, leadership best practices, managing in higher education and K12, student engagement and success, student retention, adult learning theory, adult, nontraditional, and at-risk learners, faculty retention, hiring practices, faculty burn-out, best practices in online learning, emerging technology in course design and instruction, online education, learning styles, diversity leadership, virtuous leadership, and the Community of Inquiry Framework.

Contact

Email:
lisamarieportugal@msn.com

Website:
http://drlisamarieportugal.weebly.com

Website:
https://drlisamarieportugal.wixsite.com/leadershiparchitect

References

Afeltra, A., Abbate, A., Valentini, G., & Giacomelli, R. (2019). Inflammation and dysmetabolism in systemic autoimmune diseases. *Journal of Immunology Research, 2019.*

Afzal, A., & Gauthier, J. B. (2017). Project management and practitioners in the health sector: From the Quebec healthcare system perspective to PM literature review. https://hal.archives-ouvertes.fr/hal-01579996/document

American Autoimmune Related Diseases Association Inc. (AARDA). (2020). *Autoimmune disease.* https://www.aarda.org/NEWS-INFORMATION/STATISTICS/#:~:text=Autoimmune%20Disease...%201%20Symptoms%20cross%20many%20specialties%20and,outside%20their%20own%20specialty%20area.%20More%20items...%20

Bartholomew, L. K., Markham, C. M., Ruiter, R. A. C., Fernàndez, M. E., Kok, G., & Parcel, G. S. (2016). *Planning health promotion programs: An Intervention Mapping approach* (4th ed.). Wiley.

Bergman, J. (2015, April 15). *Auto immune disease 2015.* https://www.slideshare.net/johnbchiro/auto-immune-disease-2015

Center for Natural and Integrative Medicine (CNIM). (2019). *I.V. chelation: What is chelation therapy?* https://drkalidas.com/iv-chelation/

Costello, M., Taylor, J., & O'Hara, L. (2015). Impact evaluation of a health promotion-focused organisational development strategy on a health service's capacity to deliver comprehensive primary health care. *Australian Journal of Primary Health, 21*(4), 444-449. https://doi.org/10.1071/PY14107

cs@carbswitch.com (2015, February 9). *What is autoimmune disease.* https://carbswitch.com/2015/02/09/what-is-autoimmune-disease

Daivam Wellness (2019, October 16). *When was the last time your doctor asked you to take a metal toxicity test?* https://www.daivamwellness.com/when-was-the-last-time-your-doctor-asked-you-to-take-a-metal-toxicity-test/

DrJockers.com (n.d.). *The 7 major factors causing autoimmune conditions.* https://drjockers.com/7-factors-causing-autoimmune-conditions/

Duan, L., Rao, X., & Sigdel, K. R. (2019). Regulation of inflammation in autoimmune disease. *Journal of Immunology Research, 2019*.

Fernandez, M. E., Ruiter, R. A. C., Markham, C. M., & Kok, G. (2019). Intervention mapping: Theory and evidence-based health promotion program planning: Perspective and examples. *Frontiers in Public Health, 7*, 209. https://www.frontiersin.org/article/10.3389/fpubh.2019.00209

Five Seasons Functional Medicine. (2019). *What is intestinal permeability (leaky gut)?* https://fiveseasonsmedical.com/leaky-gut/

Fontes, M., & Stawicki, M. (n.d.). *Natural medicine and detox.* https://naturalmedicineanddetox.com/

Frieden, T. R. (2010). A framework for public health action: The health impact pyramid. *American Journal of Public Health, 100*(4), 590-595.

Genetic and Rare Diseases Information Center (GARD). (2017, April 28). Heavy metal poisoning. *National Center for Advancing Translational Sciences.* https://rarediseases.info.nih.gov/diseases/6577/heavy-metal-poisoning

Gotter, A., & Murrell, D. (2018, December 13). Heavy metal poisoning. *Healthline Media.* https://www.healthline.com/health/heavy-metal-poisoning

Goudet, S., Murira, Z., Torlesse, H., Hatchard, J., & Busch-Hallen, J. (2018, November 29). Effectiveness of programme approaches to improve the coverage of maternal nutrition interventions in South Asia. *Maternal and Child Nutrition, 14*(54), e12699. https://doi.org/10.1111/mcn.12699

Grant, A., Bugge, C., & Wells, M. (2020, November 27). Designing process evaluations using case study to explore the context of complex interventions evaluated in trials. *Trials, 21*(982). https://doi.org/10.1186/s13063-020-04880-4

Hester, J., Auerbach, J., Seeff, L., Wheaton, J., Brusuelas, K., & Singleton, C. (2016). *CDC's 6|18 Initiative: Accelerating evidence into action.* https://nam.edu/wp-content/uploads/2016/05/CDCs-618-Initiative-Accelerating-Evidence-into-Action.pdf

Jones, T., (2016, May 31) Outcome measurement in nursing: Imperatives, Ideals, history, and challenges. *The Online Journal of Issues in Nursing, 21*(2). http://ojin.nursingworld.org/MainMenuCategories/ANAMarketplace/ANAPeriodicals/OJIN/TableofContents/Vol-21-2016/No2-May-2016/Outcome-Measurement-in-Nursing.html

Kim, J-J., Kim, Y-S., & Kumar, V. (2019). Heavy metal toxicity: An update of chelating therapeutic strategies. *Journal of Trace Elements in Medicine and Biology, 54*, 226-231. https://doi.org/10.1016/j.jtemb.2019.05.003.

Kok, G., Gottlieb, N. H., Peters, G. J. Y., Mullen, P. D., Parcel, G. S., Ruiter, R. A. C., Fernández, M. E., Markham, C., & Bartholomew, L. K. (2016). A Taxonomy of behavior change methods: An intervention mapping approach. *Health Psychology Review, 10*(3), 297-312. https://www.tandfonline.com/doi/full/10.1080/17437199.2015.1077155

Konijeti, G. G., Kim, N., Lewis, J. D., Groven, S., Chandrasekaran, A., Grandhe, S., Diamant, C., Singh, E., Oliveira, G., Wang, X., Molparia, B., & Torkamani, A., (2017, November 1). Efficacy of the autoimmune protocol diet for inflammatory bowel disease. *Inflammatory Bowel Diseases, 23*(11), 2054–2060. https://doi.org/10.1097/MIB.0000000000001221

Lewis, S. R. (2017). The practice of health program evaluation. *Health Promotion Practice, 18*(6), 782-784. https://doi.org/10.1177/1524839917711185

Long, H., Wang, X., Chen, Y., Wang, L., Zhao, M., & Lu, Q. (2018, August 1). Dysregulation of microRNAs in autoimmune diseases: Pathogenesis, biomarkers and potential therapeutic targets. *Cancer Letters, 428*, 90-103.

Maja, J. (2019, April 10). *How amalgam (and heavy metals) can cause Hashimoto and other autoimmune diseases.* https://www.joannamaja.com/how-amalgam-and-heavy-metals-can-cause-hashimoto-and-other-autoimmune-diseases/

Mcleod, B. (n.d.). *Introduction to intervention mapping - PowerPoint PPT presentation.* https://www.slideserve.com/benedict/introduction-to-intervention-mapping

Milne, L. (2009, June 25). *Needs assessment.* https://www.slideshare.net/lynda.milne/needs-assessment-1638514

MIT Department of Biology. (20196). *Cell biology.* https://biology.mit.edu/faculty-and-research/areas-of-research/cell-biology/

National Institute of Allergy and Infectious Disease (NIAID). (2017, May 2). *Autoimmune diseases.* https://www.niaid.nih.gov/diseases-conditions/autoimmune-diseases

National Institute of Environmental Health Sciences (NIEHS). (2020, May 6). *Autoimmune diseases.*

https://www.niehs.nih.gov/health/topics/conditions/autoimmune/index.cfm

Osborne, V., & Anderson, P. (2007, January 15). Chelation and IV nutrient therapy. *Naturopathic Doctor News & Review.* https://ndnr.com/cardiopulmonary-medicine/chelation-and-iv-nutrient-therapy/

Rayman, M. P. (2019, February). Multiple nutritional factors and thyroid disease, with particular reference to autoimmune thyroid disease. *The Proceedings of the Nutrition Society, 78*(1), 34-44.

Redoubt News LLC & Granny Good Food (2017, July 7). *Gluten intolerance is really GLYPHOSATE POISONING.* https://redoubtnews.com/2017/07/gluten-monsanto-glyphosate-poisoning/

Revived Life Health and Wellness. (n.d.). *Leaky gut: What is leaky gut.* https://revivedlife.net/leaky-gut/

Sharma, S., van Teijlingen, E., Belizán, J. M., Hundley, V., Simkhada, P., & Sicuri, E. (2016, May 23). Measuring what works: An impact evaluation of women's groups on maternal health uptake in rural Nepal. *PLoS ONE 11*(5), e0155144. https://doi.org/10.1371/journal.pone.0155144

Speziale, G. (2015, March). Strategic management of a healthcare organization: Engagement, behavioural indicators, and clinical performance, *European Heart Journal Supplements, 17,* Issue supplement A, A3-A7. https://doi.org/10.1093/eurheartj/suv003

Tringali-Health.com (2020). *Major Autohemotherapy (MAH) IV Therapy*. https://tringali-health.com/major-autohemotherapy/

Disclaimer: The content of this book is based on research conducted by Dr. Lisa Marie Portugal, unless otherwise noted. The information is presented for educational purposes only and is not intended to diagnose or prescribe for any medical or psychological condition, nor to prevent, treat, mitigate or cure such conditions. The information contained herein is not intended to replace a one-on-one relationship with a doctor or qualified healthcare professional. Therefore, this information is not intended as medical advice, but rather a sharing of knowledge and information based on research and experience. This book and Dr. Lisa Marie Portugal encourages you to make your own health care decisions based on your judgment and research in partnership with a qualified healthcare professional. These statements have not been evaluated by the Food and Drug Administration. The information in this book is not intended to diagnose, treat, cure, or prevent any disease. I am not diagnosing, prescribing, advising, or practicing medicine. I am merely presenting information for you to review, research, and consider. In addition, I receive no money or endorse any products or services listed in this book. My mother and I have used many of the services listed in the Chelation section with our naturopathy and Traditional Chinese Medicine doctors at our holistic clinic. Seek medical advice and service from your doctor or medical practitioner. You and only you are responsible if you choose to do anything based on what you read.

www.ingramcontent.com/pod-product-compliance
Lightning Source LLC
Chambersburg PA
CBHW040238220526
45473CB00001B/287